I May Be Small But I Got

My First Visit to the Dentist

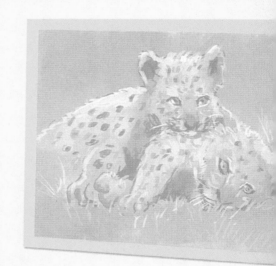

By Rose O. Wadenya, DMD   Illustrated by Sonnaz

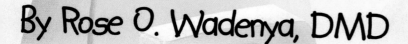

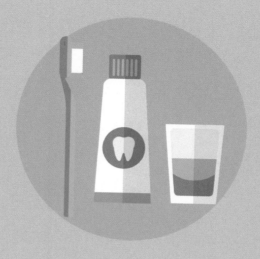

A friendly note to parents - as soon as babies are able to grab a toothbrush, they fight to brush their teeth. The reality is that kids don't develop the manual dexterity needed to brush their teeth efficiently until about age seven. Parents need to brush and then, as their kids get older, assist them in brushing and flossing until they are able to do a good job by themselves.

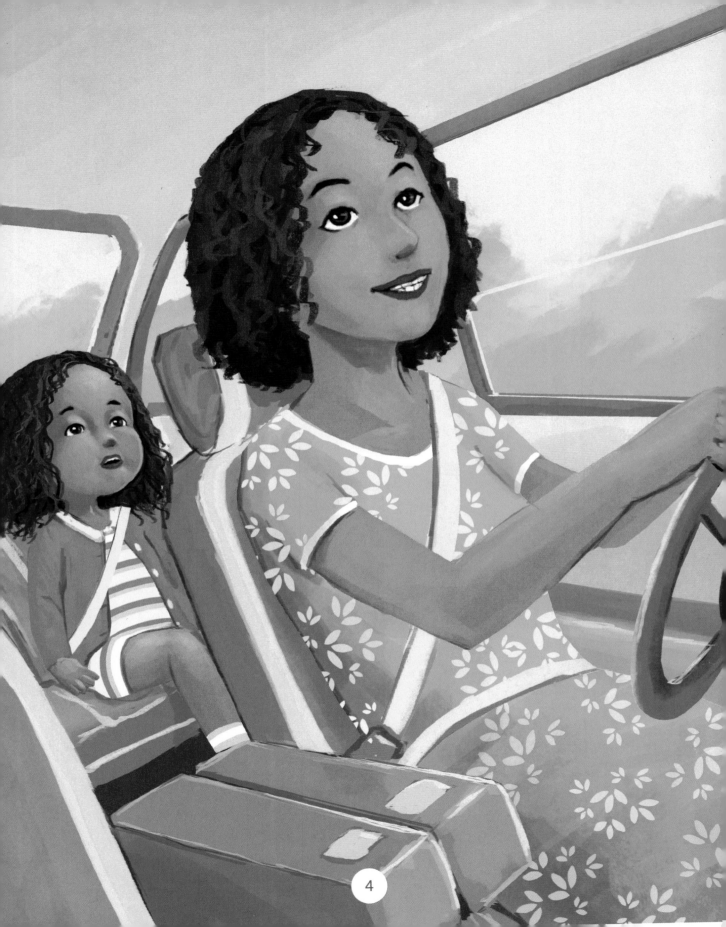

4

Today Rosie is visiting the dentist for the first time. "What if it hurts, Mommy?" Rosie is too worried to smile.

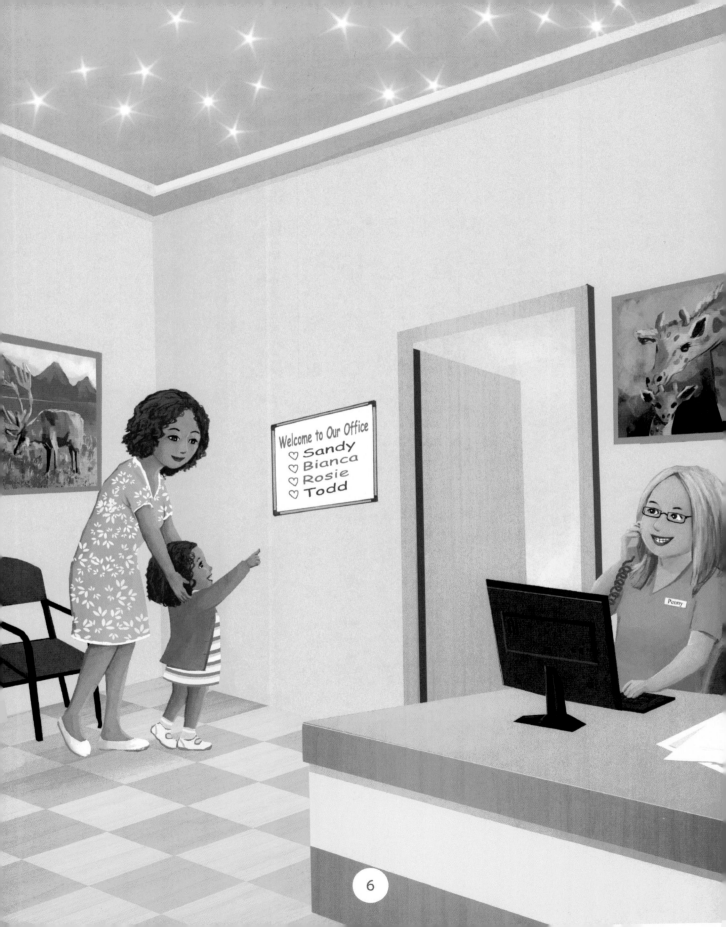

Welcome to Our Office
♡ Sandy
♡ Bianca
♡ Rosie
♡ Todd

Penny

"Look, Mommy,
that's *my* name!" she grins.
"Yes, they are expecting you,"
her mother says.

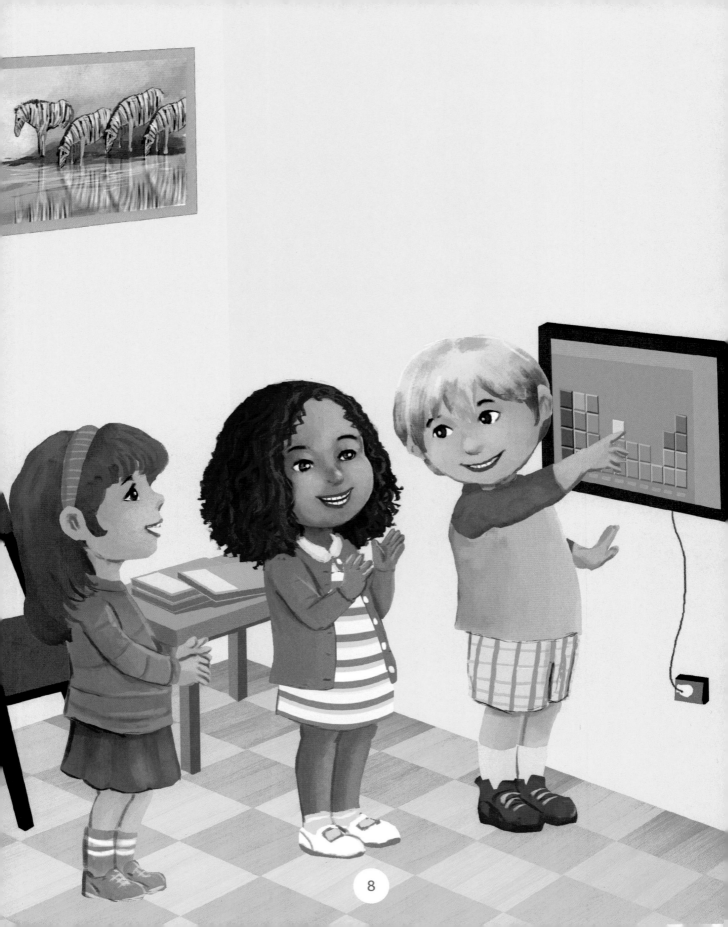

Rosie feels special now and joins the other children at the game-station. She's making new friends already!

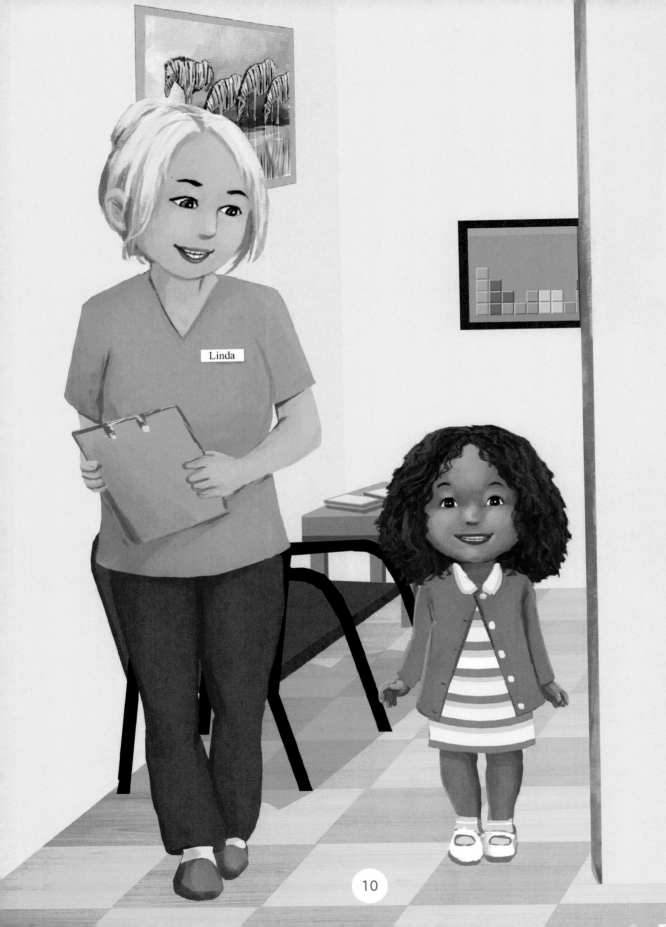

Soon it is Rosie's turn
to sit in the dental chair.
"I will show you all the cool
stuff in our office,"
says Linda, the dental hygienist.

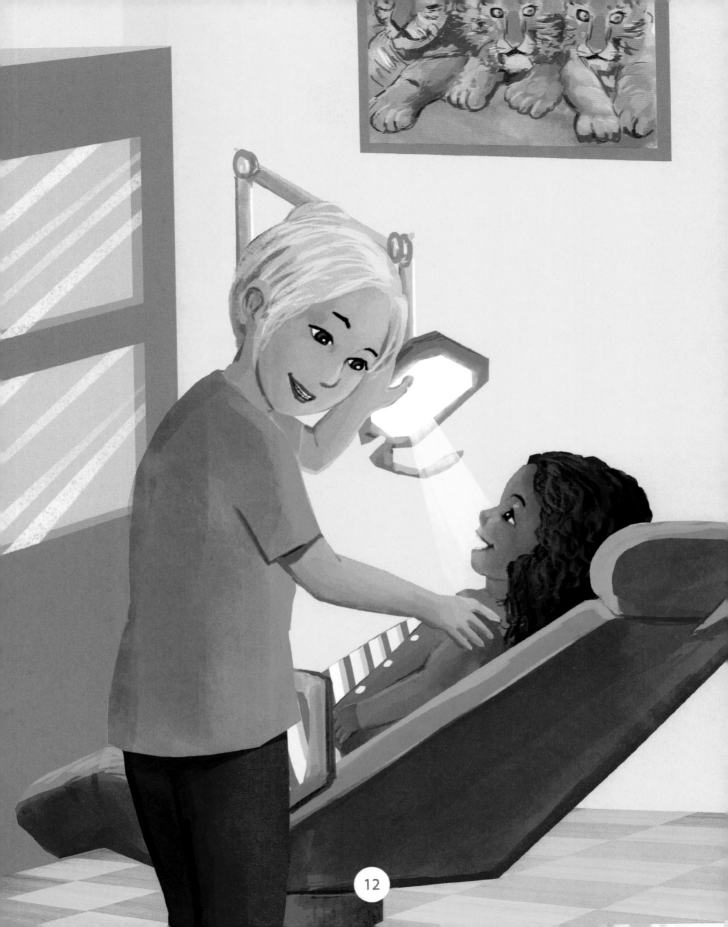

"Wow! This chair looks like a
spaceship," says Rosie.
The chair goes up then
tilts backwards.
A small bright light above
the chair shines
like a super-powerful spotlight.

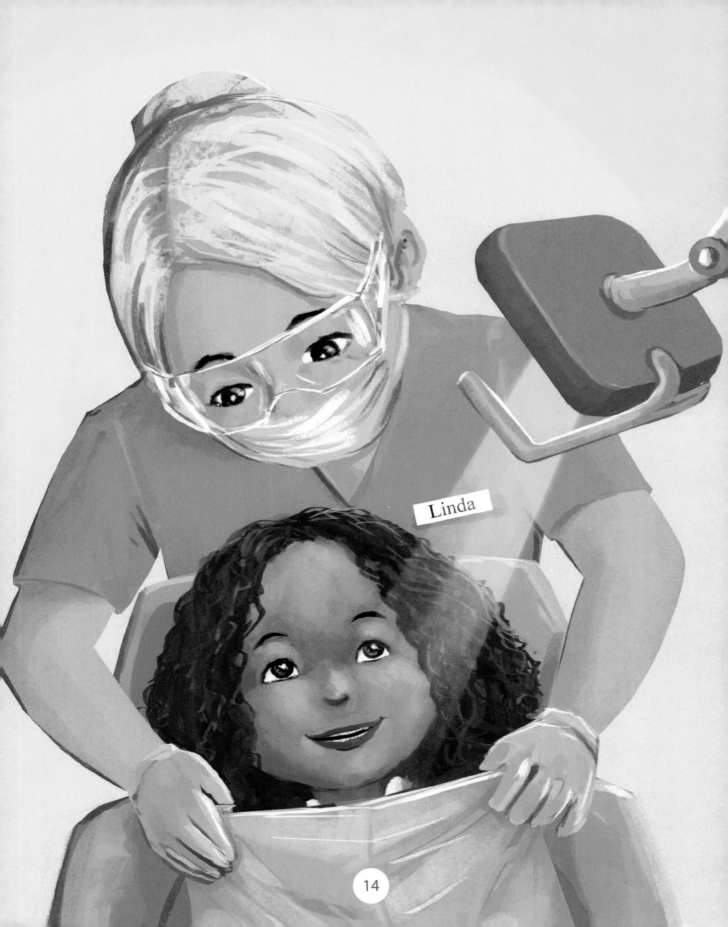

Linda puts on a mask,
gloves, and glasses.
"My gloves and mask
stop germs spreading
from me to you or
you to me," she says.
"And this paper napkin
keeps your pretty dress
from getting wet!"

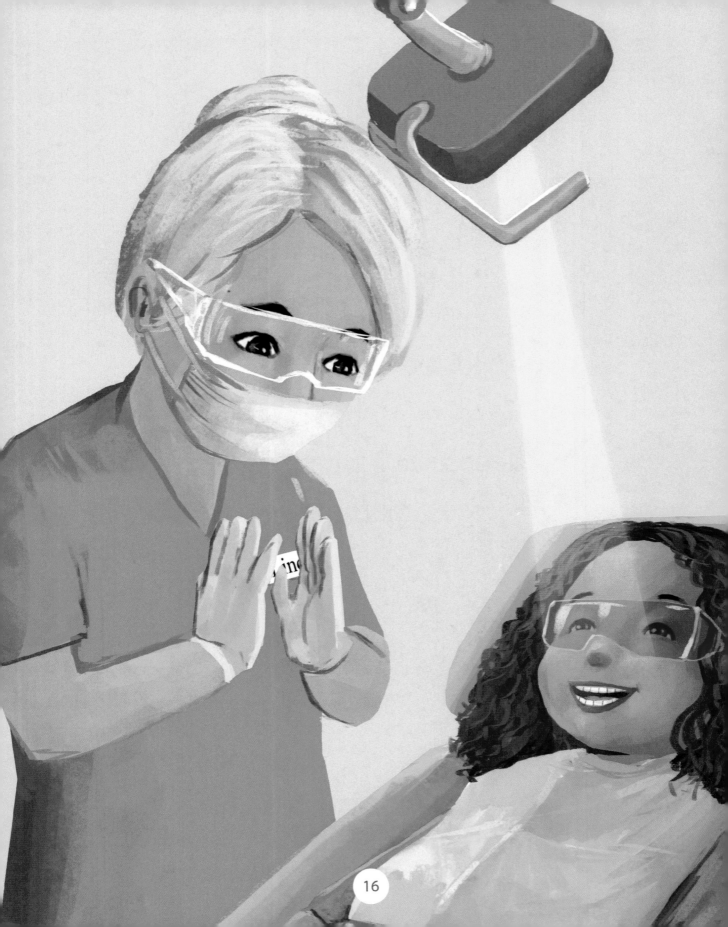

"What does that light do?"
Rosie asks curiously.
"This light helps us see all the hidden
places inside your mouth. You can wear
these sunglasses to
keep the bright light
from shining in your eyes."

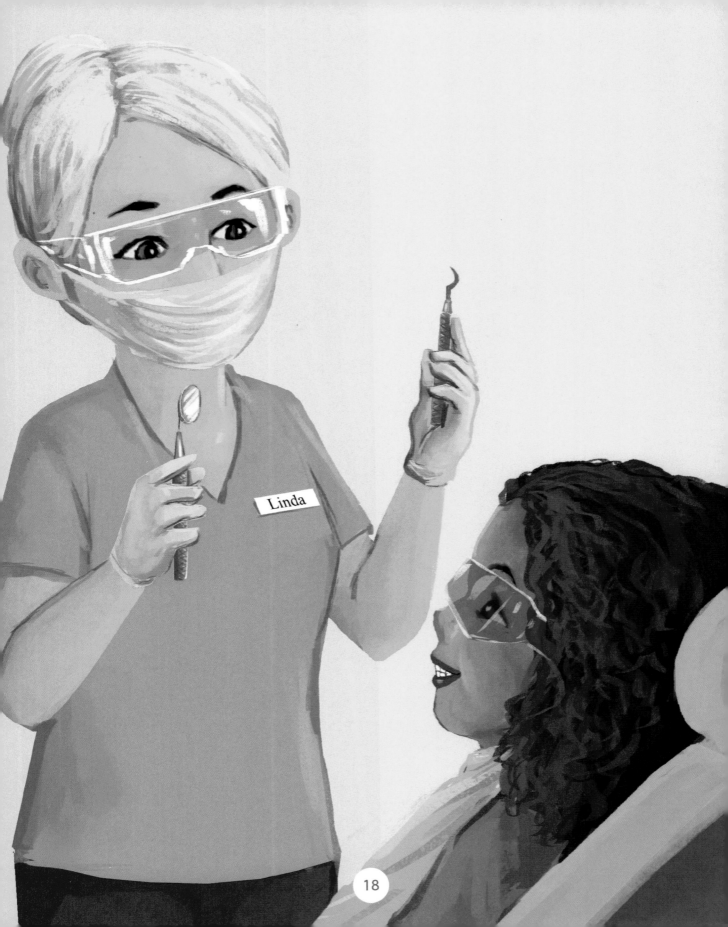

Linda shows Rosie two dentist tools;
an *explorer* and a *mirror*.
"We use these tools
to check for cavities
or holes in your teeth," she says.

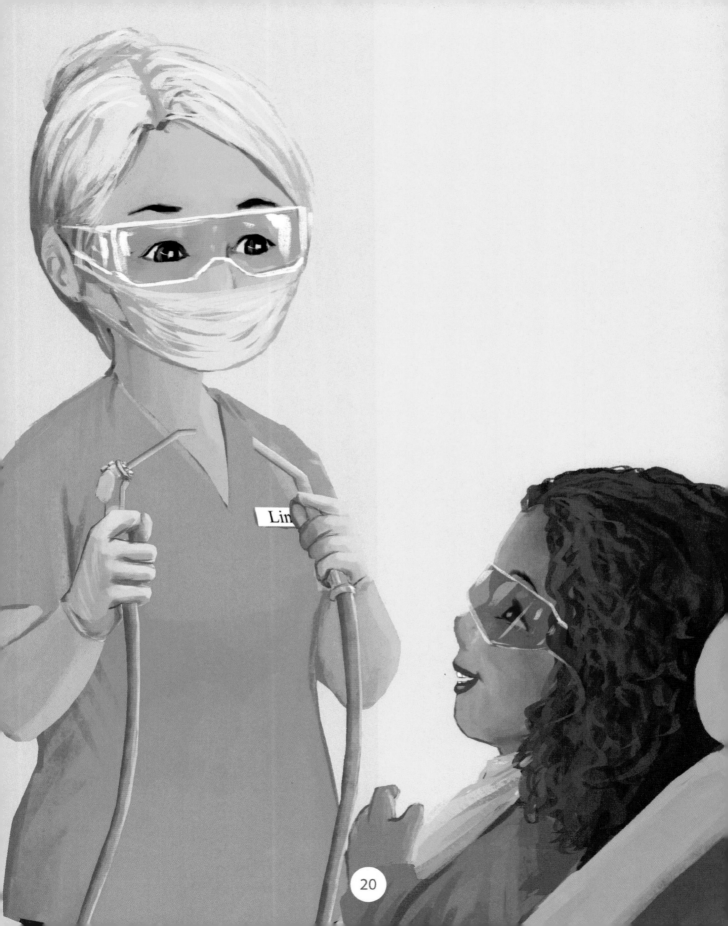

"This is our water-sprayer.
It sprays water into your mouth to
wash off any toothpaste.
But we can't work on your
teeth when your mouth is full of water,
so we have Mister Thirsty
to help us. He is like a vacuum-cleaner
that sucks up all the water, spit,
and toothpaste from your mouth."

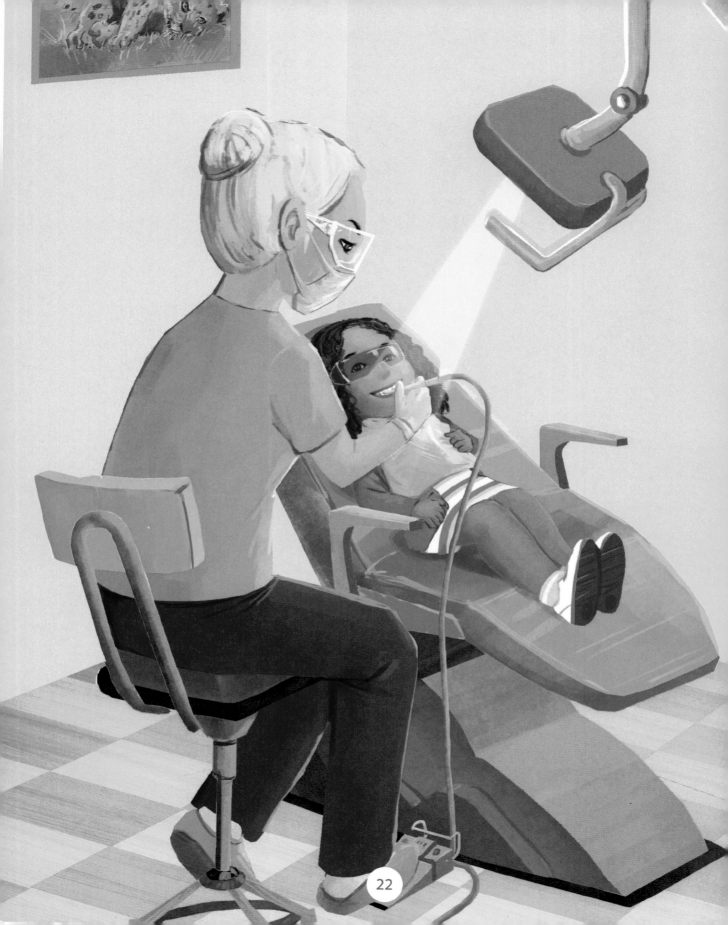

"This is a special
toothbrush that cleans
your teeth, just like
an electric toothbrush.
The toothpaste we use will make your
teeth sparkle, you'll see!"
Linda steps on a pedal
and the toothbrush begins to spin.
Rosie giggles as it
tickles her teeth!

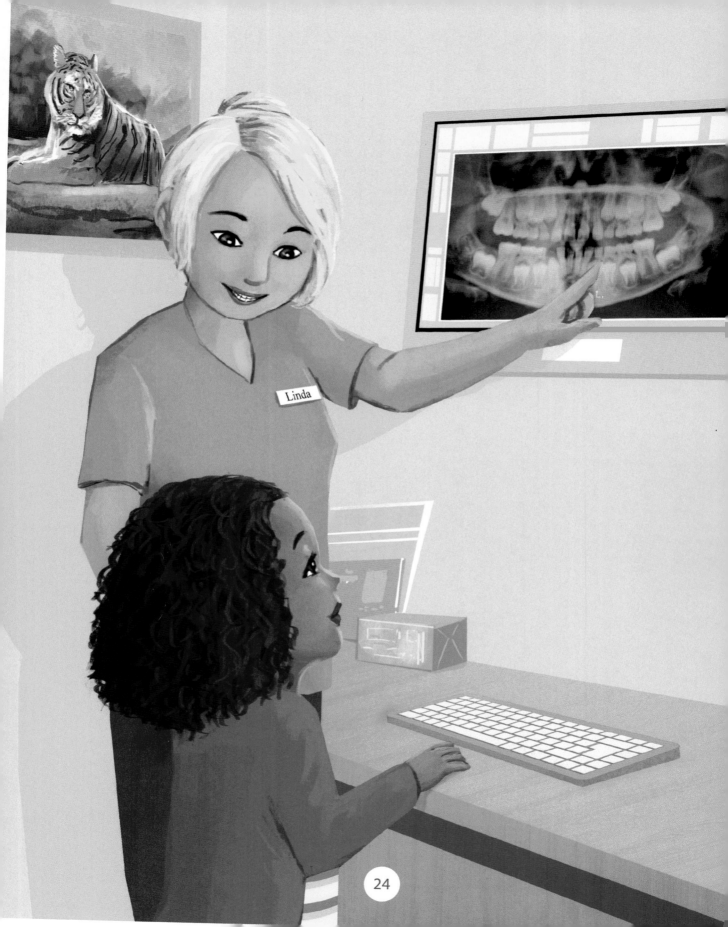

The cleaning does not take long.
Soon it is time to take
an X-ray of Rosie's teeth.
"What is an X-ray for?" Rosie asks.
"It helps us see parts of your teeth
that are hidden," says Linda.
"It works like a camera!"

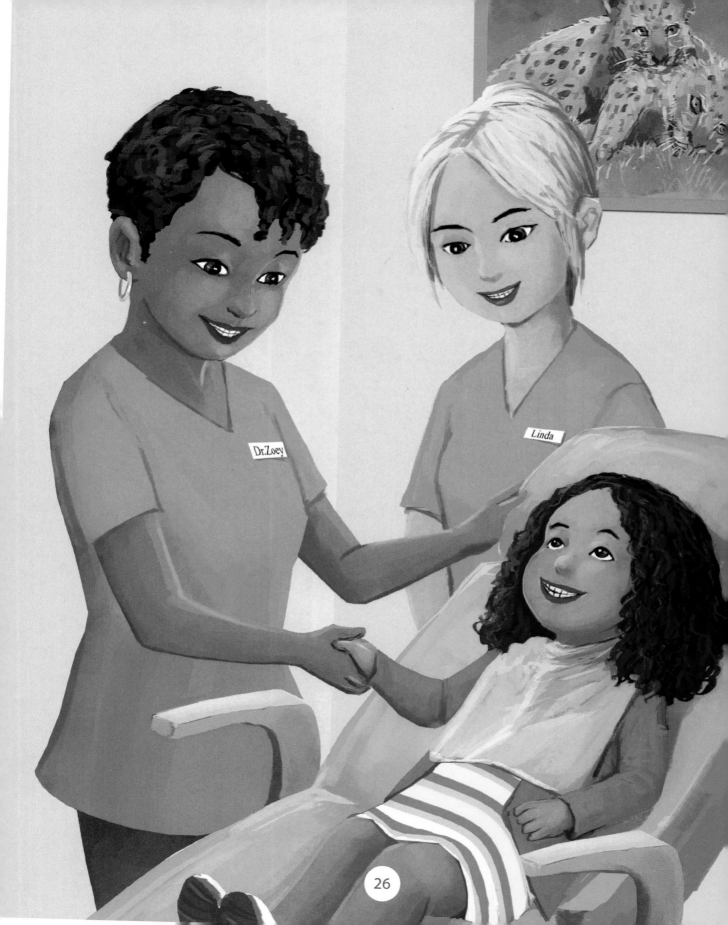

"Hi, Rosie! My name is Doctor Zoey. I am going to check your teeth to make sure everything is okay." Doctor Zoey also puts on a mask, gloves, and glasses. Rosie can see her warm smile in her eyes.

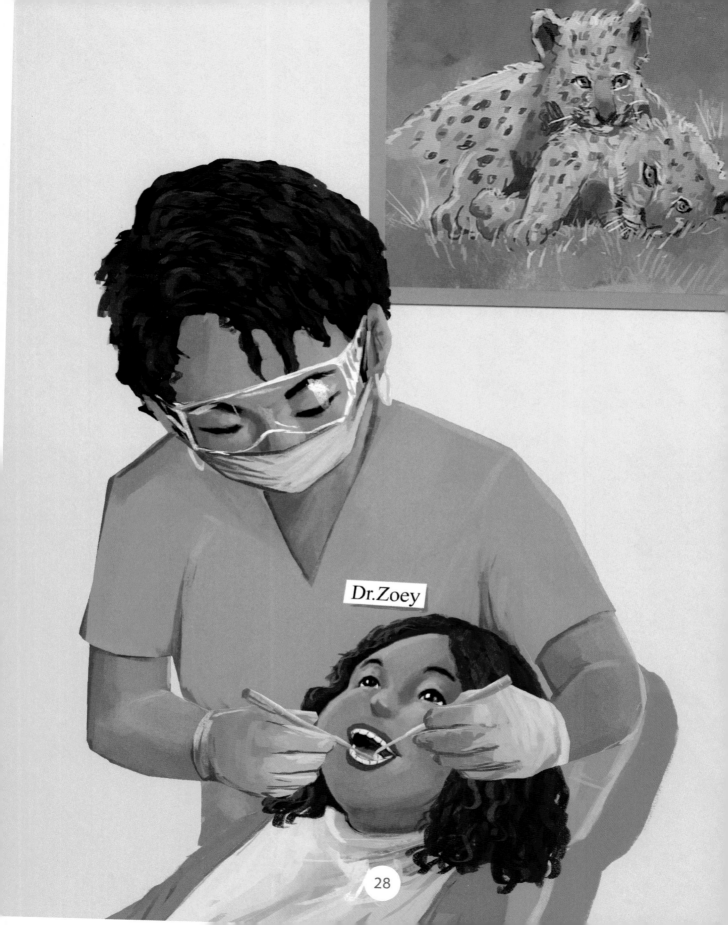

"Open wide, Rosie!"
She counts Rosie's teeth
and checks for cavities.
"Oh my, you have beautiful teeth.
Someone is doing a *great* job brushing
and flossing! Is it you, Rosie?"
Rosie smiles. "Yes, but my
Mommy helps me."
"That is great, Rosie. Keep it up!"

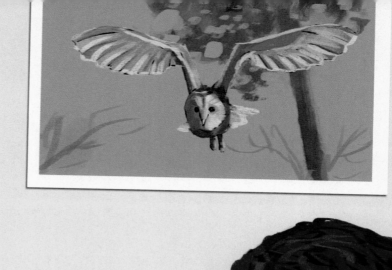

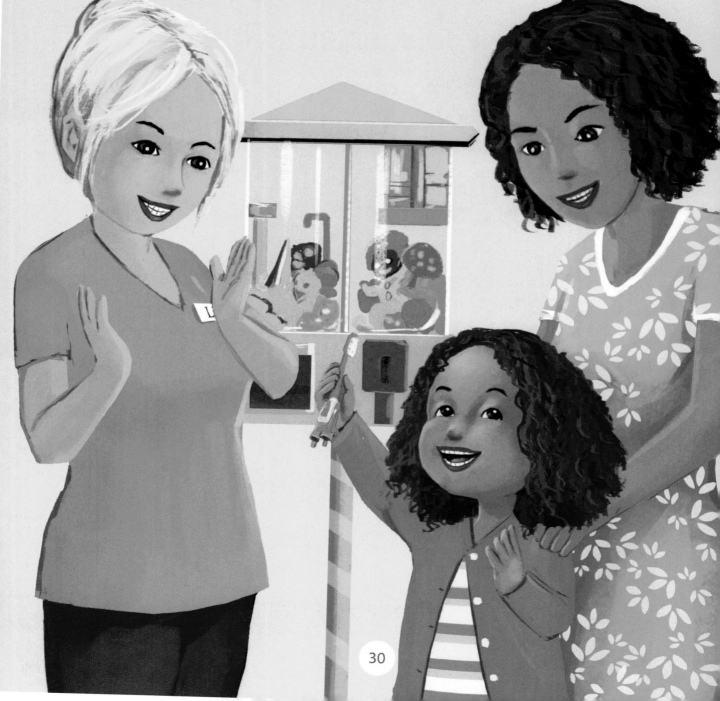

"Awesome! *Way to go, Rosie!*" says Linda.
"Are you ready for your prize?"
"Wow, I get to choose from the prize tower?
But what will I choose?
There are glowing balls,
a stretchy man... *hmm...*
I think I will take
a space-rocket toothbrush.
Thank you!" says Rosie happily.

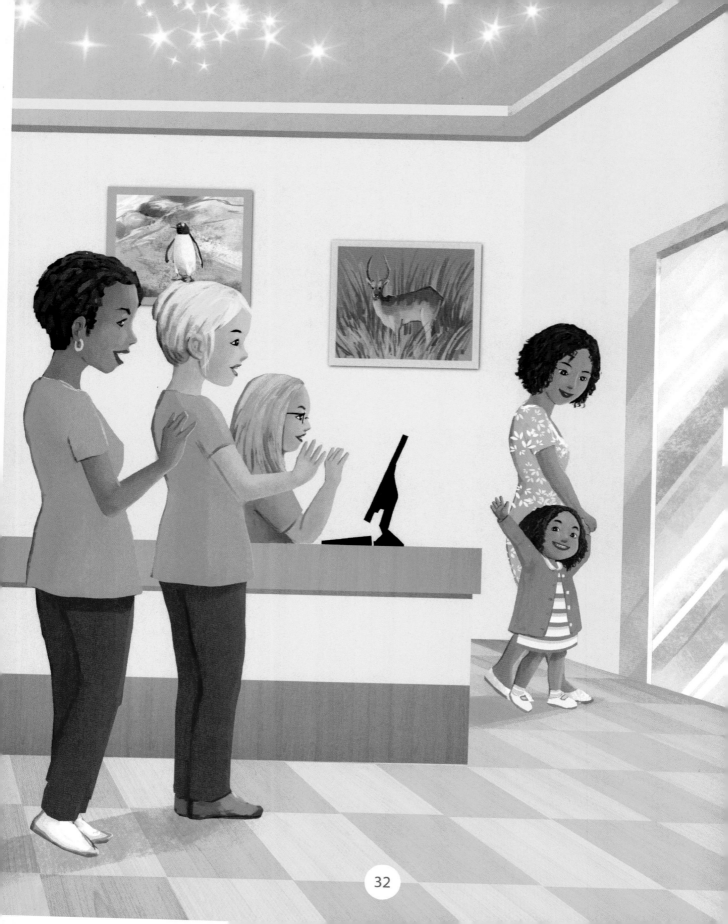

"Mommy, they are really
nice at the dentist office.
I can't wait to come back!"
says Rosie. "Your first
trip to the dentist turned
out great!" her mother smiles.

The End

A chart for My Teeth.

Parents - this chart shows us which teeth erupt and then shed at different ages in a child's development.

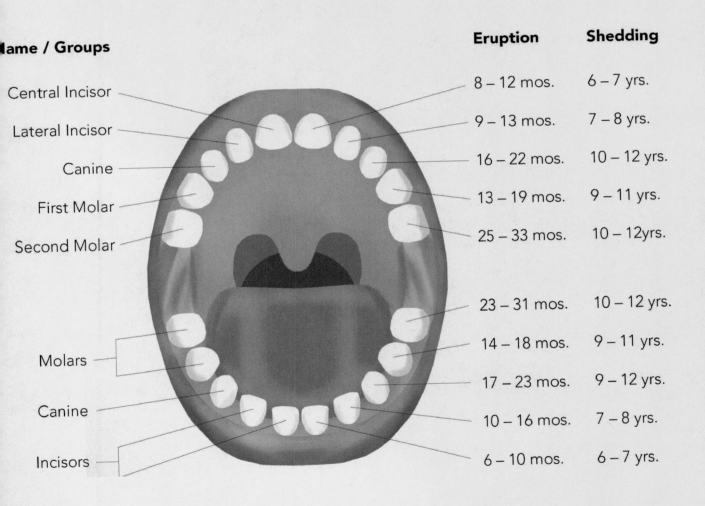

Name / Groups	Eruption	Shedding
Central Incisor	8 – 12 mos.	6 – 7 yrs.
Lateral Incisor	9 – 13 mos.	7 – 8 yrs.
Canine	16 – 22 mos.	10 – 12 yrs.
First Molar	13 – 19 mos.	9 – 11 yrs.
Second Molar	25 – 33 mos.	10 – 12yrs.
	23 – 31 mos.	10 – 12 yrs.
Molars	14 – 18 mos.	9 – 11 yrs.
	17 – 23 mos.	9 – 12 yrs.
Canine	10 – 16 mos.	7 – 8 yrs.
Incisors	6 – 10 mos.	6 – 7 yrs.

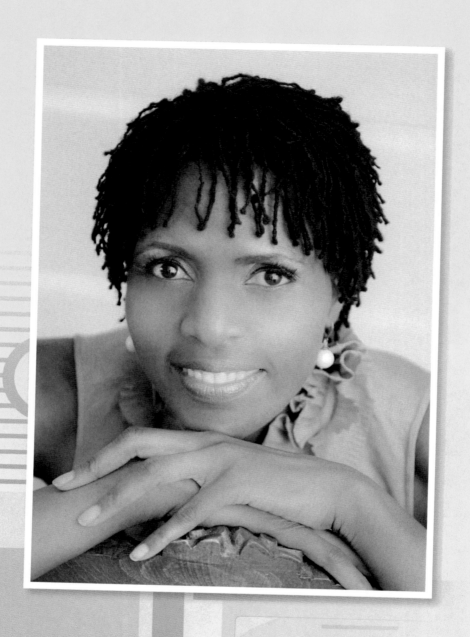

About Dr. Rose O. Wadenya

Dr. Rose O. Wadenya was born in Kenya, Africa. After college she moved to the United States where she went on to pursue her career ambitions in the healthcare industry, as well as her personal ambitions to become a writer.

Rose received her doctorate of Dental Medicine from the University of Pennsylvania where her primary interest was reducing oral diseases in children. Since then she has published widely in this area, and delivered many presentations regarding ways to improve oral healthcare for underserved children. Rose is Board Certified by the American Board of Pediatric Dentistry.

At her dental practice, Rose combines her love for storytelling and humming tunes, and uses this as a way to keep her patients intrigued and relaxed, even giddy, during treatment. In her twenty-five years of practice, she has found that this is a great solution to anxiety and worry in children during dental treatment. With her patients asking for more stories after each visit, she was inspired to write and print each of them so that they'd be readily available to all children around the world.

Rose is an author of numerous fun and witty books that aim to help children understand the importance of dental care and healthy teeth. Her books offer humorous, insightful, thought-provoking, and sometimes peculiar stories that promise to keep kids inspired about their dental health.

Ranging from animal heroes to the Tooth Fairy, teasing among youngsters to the dreaded Sugar Bugs, her wonderfully illustrated books present entirely new perspectives on teeth and issues centered on dental care for kids.

Although she'll forever be African at heart, she now lives in Havertown, Pennsylvania, with her husband and two children.

You can visit Dr. Rose's website at www.eaglecrestkids.com.

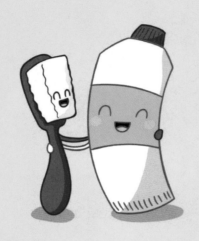

Made in the USA
Middletown, DE
16 October 2021

50439137R00022